Post-Polio Syndrome

A Beginner's 3-Step Quick Start Guide on Managing Post-Polio Syndrome Through Natural Methods and Diet, With Sample Recipes

mf

copyright © 2022 Patrick Marshwell

All rights reserved No part of this book may be reproduced, or stored in a retrieval system, or transmitted in any form or by any means, electronic, mechanical, photocopying, recording, or otherwise, without express written permission of the publisher.

Disclaimer

By reading this disclaimer, you are accepting the terms of the disclaimer in full. If you disagree with this disclaimer, please do not read the guide.

All of the content within this guide is provided for informational and educational purposes only, and should not be accepted as independent medical or other professional advice. The author is not a doctor, physician, nurse, mental health provider, or registered nutritionist/dietician. Therefore, using and reading this guide does not establish any form of a physician-patient relationship.

Always consult with a physician or another qualified health provider with any issues or questions you might have regarding any sort of medical condition. Do not ever disregard any qualified professional medical advice or delay seeking that advice because of anything you have read in this guide. The information in this guide is not intended to be any sort of medical advice and should not be used in lieu of any medical advice by a licensed and qualified medical professional.

The information in this guide has been compiled from a variety of known sources. However, the author cannot attest to or guarantee the accuracy of each source and thus should not be held liable for any errors or omissions.

You acknowledge that the publisher of this guide will not be held liable for any loss or damage of any kind incurred as a result of this guide or the reliance on any information provided within this guide. You acknowledge and agree that you assume all risk and responsibility for any action you undertake in response to the information in this guide.

Using this guide does not guarantee any particular result (e.g., weight loss or a cure). By reading this guide, you acknowledge that there are no guarantees to any specific outcome or results you can expect.

All product names, diet plans, or names used in this guide are for identification purposes only and are the property of their respective owners. The use of these names does not imply endorsement. All other trademarks cited herein are the property of their respective owners.

Where applicable, this guide is not intended to be a substitute for the original work of this diet plan and is, at most, a supplement to the original work for this diet plan and never a direct substitute. This guide is a personal expression of the facts of that diet plan.

Where applicable, persons shown in the cover images are stock photography models and the publisher has obtained the rights to use the images through license agreements with third-party stock image companies.

Table of Contents

Introduction	**6**
What Is Post-Polio Syndrome?	**8**
Causes	9
Symptoms	12
Diagnosing Post-Polio Syndrome	**15**
The 3-Step Guide on Managing Post-Polio Syndrome	**17**
Step 1 - Focus on your medications	17
Step 2 - Physical therapy	18
Step 3 - Diet and nutrition	18
7-Day Sample Meal Plan	22
Sample Recipes	**24**
Cauliflower and Mushroom Bake	25
Cucumber with Fennel and Creamy Avocado Dressing	26
Roasted Okra and Smoked Paprika	27
Spice Trade Beans and Bulgar	28
Vegan Mac and Cheese	30
Potato and Egg Salad	32
Avocado Chicken Lemon Salad	34
Guilt-Free Egg Salad	37
Prosciutto-Roast Beef Tenderloin	38
Flavored Italian Meatballs	39
Chicken Wrap (Cajun Style)	41
Slow Cooker Dairy-Free Buttered Chicken	42
Keto Taco Shells	44
One-Pot Chicken and Rice	46
Red Velvet Molten Lava Cake	48
Prevention of Post-Polio Syndrome	**50**
Post-Polio Syndrome and Quality of Life	**52**
FAQ About Post-Polio Syndrome	**54**
Key Takeaways	**57**
References and Helpful Links	**58**

Introduction

Post-polio syndrome (PPS) is a condition that affects approximately 25 to 50 percent of people who have previously had poliomyelitis (polio). Although there is no cure for PPS, there are treatments available that can help manage the symptoms and improve the quality of life.

There are three main types of treatment for PPS:

1. *Medication:* There are a variety of medications available that can assist in relieving the pain, fatigue, and muscle weakness that are associated with PPS.
2. *Physical therapy:* A person who has PPS can work with a physical therapist to develop an exercise program that is tailored to their needs and will help them improve their strength and endurance.
3. *Diet and nutrition:* People who have PPS should prioritize maintaining a healthy diet and getting the recommended amount of rest and sleep each night.

In this beginner's quick start guide, we will go over the following in great detail:

- About post-polio syndrome
- Causes and symptoms of PPS
- Diagnosing and treating PPS
- Natural ways to prevent and manage PPS
- PPS-friendly diet and meal plans

What Is Post-Polio Syndrome?

Post-polio syndrome (PPS) is a condition that affects some people who have had polio. Symptoms can include muscle weakness, pain, and fatigue. There is no cure for PPS, but there are treatments that can help manage the symptoms. Treatment options include physical therapy, occupational therapy, and lifestyle changes such as diet and exercise.

People who have had polio in the past might sometimes develop a disorder called post-polio syndrome (PPS). It is not known for certain what causes post-polio syndrome (PPS), but it is believed that it is related to the degradation of nerve cells that were caused by the poliovirus. PPS symptoms typically manifest anywhere from 15 to 30 years after the initial infection.

Weakness in the muscles is the PPS patient's most common symptom. This condition can range from somewhat moderate to quite severe, and it can affect any muscle in the body. Along with pain, other symptoms may include fatigue, sensitivity to colds, difficulty swallowing, and difficulty swallowing food.

There is no cure for PPS, but there are treatments that can help manage the symptoms. Treatment options include physical therapy, occupational therapy, and lifestyle changes such as diet and exercise. Physical therapy can help improve muscle strength and function. Occupational therapy can help with activities of daily living. Lifestyle changes such as a healthy diet and regular exercise can help improve overall health and well-being.

If you think you may have PPS, see your doctor for an evaluation. There is no one test that can diagnose PPS, so the diagnosis is made based on a review of your medical history and symptoms. There is no specific treatment for PPS, but there are many options available to help manage the symptoms. With proper management, most people with PPS can live normal, active lives.

Causes

The exact cause of PPS is unknown, but it is thought to be due to the degeneration of nerve cells that were affected by the poliovirus. Symptoms of PPS usually begin 15-30 years after the initial infection.

There are numerous potential causes of PPS; however, the degeneration of nerve cells that occurred as a result of the polio virus is the most likely explanation for this condition. The following are some additional possible causes:

- *Autoimmune reaction* - Autoimmune reactions are when the body's immune system attacks healthy cells. In the case of post-polio syndrome, it is believed that the immune system attacks the nerve cells that were damaged by the poliovirus. This damage can lead to muscle weakness and paralysis.
- *Muscle inflammation* - One possible cause of the post-polio syndrome is muscle inflammation. When muscles are inflamed, they can become weak and shrunken. This can lead to the development of new polio symptoms, even years after the initial infection has resolved. In some cases, the inflammation may be caused by an autoimmune reaction, in which the body's immune system mistakenly attacks healthy tissues.

Treatment for muscle inflammation typically includes corticosteroids or immunosuppressive drugs. However, these medications can have serious side effects, so it is important to work closely with a doctor to determine whether they are appropriate for you.

- *Joint or bone problems* - Problems with the joints or the bones are one of the possible causes of post-polio syndrome. It's possible that this is because the polio virus has the ability to attack cells in the nervous system that are in charge of controlling movement in muscles. This can result in muscle weakness and atrophy, which, in turn, can lead to problems with the joints and bones.

- *Nerve damage* - There are a number of possible causes of post-polio syndrome, but the most likely cause is nerve damage. When the original polio infection damages the nerves, it can cause long-term problems. The nerves may not be able to repair themselves properly, and this can lead to muscle weakness and wasting. In some cases, the nerves may become permanently damaged, and this can cause post-polio syndrome.

- *Polio vaccine reaction* - It is believed that post-polio syndrome is caused by a reaction to the polio vaccine. The virus that causes polio is no longer active, so the body can't build immunity to it. However, the body can still build up immunity to the components of the vaccine. When someone with post-polio syndrome comes in contact with the virus, their immune system overreacts and damages their own nerves. This can cause new symptoms, or worsen existing ones.

It is not clear what the exact cause of the post-polio syndrome is. It is thought to be related to the damage that the original polio infection causes to the nervous system. It is also believed that post-polio syndrome is caused by a reaction to the polio vaccine. The virus that causes polio is no longer active, so the body can't build up immunity to it.

However, the body can still build up immunity to the components of the vaccine. When someone with post-polio syndrome comes in contact with the virus, their immune system overreacts and damages their own nerves. This can cause new symptoms, or worsen existing ones.

Symptoms

PPS is a rare condition that can occur in people who have previously had polio. Symptoms of PPS usually begin 15-30 years after the initial infection.

The most common symptom of PPS is muscle weakness. This can range from mild to severe and can affect any muscle in the body. Other symptoms include pain, fatigue, cold intolerance, and difficulty swallowing.

- *Muscle Weakness* - The most common symptom of PPS is muscle weakness. This can range from mild to severe and can affect any muscle in your body. The cause of muscle weakness is unknown, but it is thought to be related to the damage that the disease causes to the nervous system.
- *Pain* - Pain is another common symptom of PPS. It can be caused by muscle weakness, inflammation, or joint problems. You may experience pain in your muscles, joints, or both. The pain may be mild, moderate, or severe. It may come and go, or it may be

constant. The pain may get worse with activity, or it may not.
- ***Fatigue*** - Fatigue is a common symptom of PPS. You may feel tired all the time, even if you've had a full night's sleep. Fatigue can be caused by muscle weakness, pain, or difficulty sleeping. Muscle weakness can make it hard to do your everyday activities. Pain can make it hard to sleep at night.
- ***Cold Intolerance*** - Cold intolerance is a common symptom of PPS. It can be caused by muscle weakness or nerve damage. Muscle weakness can make it difficult to move and stay warm. Nerve damage can disrupt the signals that tell your body to conserve heat. It can also cause you to feel pain when exposed to cold temperatures. If you have cold intolerance, you may need to take steps to protect yourself from the cold. This may include wearing warm clothing, avoiding drafts, and taking breaks from the cold when necessary. You may also need to stay hydrated and avoid caffeine, as both can make cold intolerance worse.
- ***Difficulty Swallowing*** - Difficulty swallowing is a common symptom of PPS. It can be caused by muscle weakness or nerve damage. The muscles that help you

swallow may be weakened, and the nerves that control those muscles may be damaged. This can make it hard for you to swallow food or liquids. You may also feel like food is stuck in your throat. Difficulty swallowing can make it hard for you to eat and drink, and it can lead to weight loss.

Diagnosing Post-Polio Syndrome

There is no single test that can diagnose PPS. Instead, doctors will use a combination of medical history, physical examination, and tests to rule out other conditions. Your doctor will ask about your medical history and symptoms and perform a physical examination. They may also order blood tests or imaging tests to rule out other conditions. If your doctor suspects PPS, they may refer you to a specialist for further evaluation.

Medical History - Your doctor will ask about your medical history in order to diagnose post-polio syndrome. This will include questions about your polio infection as well as any other illnesses you may have had since then. They will also inquire about your symptoms and the time frame during which they first appeared.

Physical Examination - Your doctor will examine you for muscle weakness and atrophy when diagnosing post-polio syndrome. They may also test your reflexes and sensation. In some cases, electromyography (EMG) may be used to help diagnose post-polio syndrome. This test measures the electrical activity of your muscles and can show which muscles are affected by the condition. If you have post-polio syndrome, EMG results may show reduced electrical activity in the affected muscles.

Tests - your doctor will likely order a combination of tests to rule out other conditions and check for signs of nerve damage. These may include blood tests, magnetic resonance imaging (MRI), and electromyography (EMG). Blood tests can help to check for inflammation, while MRI and EMG are used to assess nerve damage. In some cases, a muscle biopsy may also be ordered. This involves taking a small sample of muscle tissue for laboratory analysis.

Although there is currently no treatment available for post-polio syndrome, it is critical to diagnose it as early as possible. This can help to ensure that you get the highest quality care and treatment that is available to you.

The 3-Step Guide on Managing Post-Polio Syndrome

However, there are treatments that can help alleviate and manage the symptoms of Post-polio Syndrome (PPS). Although there is no cure for PPS, these treatments can help. Those who have PPS may also benefit from using natural treatments and changing their diet in order to improve their quality of life.

Step 1 - Focus on your medications

While there is no cure for PPS, there are a number of medications that can help relieve pain, fatigue, and muscle weakness. Pain relievers such as acetaminophen or ibuprofen can help to reduce pain and inflammation. If you are experiencing fatigue, your doctor may recommend a low-dose antidepressant or a stimulant such as modafinil. For muscle weakness, treatments such as physical therapy, occupational therapy, and exercise can be helpful. In some cases, your doctor may also prescribe corticosteroids or other immunosuppressive medications.

Step 2 - Physical therapy

One of the most important treatments for PPS is physical therapy. A physical therapist can design an exercise program specifically for people with PPS that will help improve strength and endurance. In addition, PT can also help to stretch tight muscles and reduce inflammation. Other treatments for PPS include occupational therapy, speech therapy, and orthopedic devices.

Step 3 - Diet and nutrition

Eating a healthy diet is important for everyone, but it's especially important for people with PPS. Eating a balanced diet that includes plenty of fruits, vegetables, and whole grains can help to boost your energy and reduce fatigue. In addition, drinking plenty of fluids and getting enough rest are also important for managing PPS.

Sensible Diet

Following a sensible diet can help improve the symptoms of post-polio syndrome. The main goals of your nutritional plan should be:

- to increase the amount of protein
- increase the number of calories
- avoid empty calories, and;
- cut back on alcohol.

Muscle tissue is the largest consumer of protein in the body, so it is important for polio survivors to have a generous amount of protein in their diet.

This can be achieved by eating:

- lean meat
- nuts
- fish
- eggs, and;
- oatmeal

It is also important to drink plenty of fluids, especially water. The results of following a sensible diet should be an improvement in symptoms, increased energy, and faster recovery from overworked muscles.

Foods to Avoid

There are certain foods that can worsen the symptoms of PPS and should be avoided. These include:

- *Sugary foods* - for example, candy, cookies, cake, and ice cream.
- *High-fat foods* - for example, greasy hamburgers, and french fries.
- *Alcohol* - drinking alcohol can increase fatigue and muscle weakness.
- *Caffeine* - caffeinated beverages can worsen symptoms of fatigue.

- ***Processed foods*** - these foods are often high in sugar and unhealthy fats.

If you have PPS, it is important to talk to your doctor about the best diet for you. They may recommend that you see a registered dietitian who can help you create a healthy eating plan.

In conclusion, post-polio syndrome is a serious condition that requires proper diagnosis and treatment. While there is no cure for PPS, treatments such as medications, physical therapy, and occupational therapy can help to improve symptoms and quality of life. In addition, eating a healthy diet and getting enough rest are also important for managing PPS. If you have PPS, be sure to talk to your doctor about the best treatment options for you.

In addition to these treatments, people who have PPS can also do a number of other things to help manage their symptoms and improve their overall quality of life. These are the following:

1. **Pace yourself**

    People with PPS often find that their symptoms get worse after periods of activity. As a result, it is important to pace yourself and avoid overexertion. This means taking frequent rests, setting realistic goals, and breaking up activities into smaller chunks.

By doing this, you can help to minimize the impact of PPS on your life.

2. **Conserve your energy**

   There is no cure for PPS, but there are a number of ways to manage the condition and improve your quality of life. One of the most important things you can do is to conserve your energy. This means sitting down when possible, using assistive devices, and avoiding excessive heat or cold. By conserving your energy, you will be able to do the things you enjoy for longer periods of time.

3. **Stay active**

   It is important to stay as active as possible, even if it means modifying your activities. Regular exercise can help improve strength and endurance, and can also help reduce pain and fatigue. If you have Post-Polio Syndrome, it is important to talk to your doctor about an exercise program that is right for you. In some cases, physical therapy may also be recommended.

4. **Stay connected**

   There is no one-size-fits-all approach to managing post-polio syndrome (PPS). However, there are a few general tips that may be helpful in dealing with the condition. One of which is to stay connected with others who have PPS. There are a number of support groups available for people with PPS, and talking with others who understand what you are going through can be helpful in dealing with the challenges of the condition.

5. **Take care of yourself**

    Taking care of yourself both physically and emotionally is important for dealing with PPS. This includes eating a healthy diet, getting regular exercise, and getting adequate rest and sleep. It is also important to find ways to relax and reduce stress in your life.

Post-polio syndrome is a condition that can be managed effectively with the right treatments and lifestyle changes. By pacing yourself, staying active, and taking care of yourself both physically and emotionally, you can improve your quality of life despite having PPS.

7-Day Sample Meal Plan

Following a weekly meal will greatly benefit you in sticking to eating healthier meals. Here is a sample meal plan made for a week that you can either follow or modify accordingly. The meals listed below are lifted from the sample recipes included in this guide. The purpose of creating a meal plan is to help you to watch what you are about to consume and make sure you're meeting your daily nutrition needs.

Meal	Breakfast	Lunch	Dinner
Day 1	Cauliflower and Mushroom Bake	Vegan Mac and Cheese	Slow Cooker Dairy-Free Buttered Chicken
Day 2	Avocado Chicken Lemon Salad	Cucumber with Fennel and Creamy Avocado Dressing	Chicken Wrap (Cajun Style)
Day 3	Vegan Mac and Cheese	Flavored Italian Meatballs	Spice Trade Beans and Bulgar
Day 4	Roasted Okra and Smoked Paprika	Keto Taco Shells	Prosciutto-Roast Beef Tenderloin
Day 5	Potato and Egg Salad	One-Pot Chicken and Rice	Potato and Egg Salad
Day 6	Guilt-Free Egg Salad	Chicken Wrap (Cajun Style)	Avocado Chicken Lemon Salad
Day 7	Red Velvet Molten Lava Cake	Cauliflower and Mushroom Bake	Prosciutto-Roast Beef Tenderloin

Sample Recipes

Cauliflower and Mushroom Bake

Ingredients:

- 3 cups cauliflower florets
- 1 cup fresh mushroom, chopped
- 1/2 cup red onion, chopped
- 1/3 cup green onion, chopped
- 2 garlic cloves, finely chopped
- 2 tsp. apple cider vinegar
- 2 tsp. lemon juice
- 1/2 tsp. salt
- 1/4 tsp. pepper*
- 1 tbsp. olive oil

Instructions:

1. Preheat the oven to 350°F. Lightly grease a baking pan.
2. Combine red onion, cauliflower, olive oil, garlic, mushroom, apple cider vinegar, lemon juice, salt, and pepper in a bowl. Mix well.
3. Pour the mixture into the greased baking pan.
4. Place inside the oven and bake for 45 minutes. Stir.
5. When vegetables are golden brown and tender, remove them from the oven.
6. Garnish with green onions. Serve and enjoy.

*black pepper may be substituted with white pepper

Cucumber with Fennel and Creamy Avocado Dressing

Ingredients:

- 2 cups sliced cucumber
- 1/2 medium avocado, peeled and pit discarded
- 1/4 tsp. and a dash salt
- freshly ground black pepper, to taste
- 2 tbsp. fresh lemon juice
- 1 large fennel, outer layer removed
- 1 tbsp. finely chopped chives

Instructions:

1. In a large bowl, combine cucumber and fennel.
2. Toss with 1/4 tsp. of salt and pepper. Set aside.
3. In a food processor, combine avocado and lemon juice. Process until smooth for about 20 seconds.
4. Add the avocado mixture to the cucumber mixture. Combine thoroughly.
5. Add chives and a dash of salt.
6. Serve and enjoy at once.

Roasted Okra and Smoked Paprika

Ingredients:

- 1/2 tsp. pepper
- 1/4 tsp. garlic powder
- 1-1/2 tsp. smoked paprika
- 3 lb. fresh okra pods
- 3/4 tsp. salt
- 3 tbsp. lemon juice
- 3 tbsp. olive oil

Instructions:

1. Preheat the oven to 400°F.
2. Toss together all ingredients.
3. Arrange them in a baking pan.
4. Roast okra until they are lightly browned and tender.
5. Serve and enjoy.

Spice Trade Beans and Bulgar

Ingredients:

- 1 can 14-1/2 oz. diced tomatoes, undrained
- 1 can 15 oz. garbanzo beans or chickpeas, rinsed and drained
- 1 can 28 oz. crushed tomatoes
- 1 carton 32 oz. vegetable broth
- 1 medium sweet red pepper, chopped
- 1 tbsp. ground cumin
- 1 tbsp. paprika
- 1 tsp. pepper
- 1/2 cup golden raisins
- 1/2 tsp. cayenne pepper
- 1/2 tsp. ground cinnamon
- 1-1/2 cups bulgur
- 2 medium onions, chopped
- 2 tbsp. brown sugar
- 2 tbsp. soy sauce
- 2 tsp. ground ginger
- 3 tbsp. canola oil, divided
- 5 garlic cloves, minced
- optional: minced fresh cilantro

Instructions:

1. In a large skillet, heat 2 tbsp. oil over medium-high heat.

2. Add onions and pepper; cook and stir until tender.
3. Add garlic and seasonings.
4. Transfer to a 5-qt. slow cooker.
5. In the same skillet, heat the remaining oil over medium-high heat.
6. Add bulgur. Cook and stir until lightly browned.
7. Add tomatoes, broth, brown sugar, and soy sauce to the slow cooker.
8. Cover and cook on low for 3-4 hours or until bulgur is tender.
9. Stir in beans and raisins. Cook for 30 minutes longer.
10. If desired, sprinkle with cilantro upon serving.

Vegan Mac and Cheese

Ingredients:

- 2 cups water
- 8 baby carrots
- 1 sweet potato, peeled and chopped
- 1/2 of a sweet onion, chopped
- 1 zucchini, peeled and chopped
- 12 oz. of pasta, cook according to packaging

Cheese sauce:

- boiled vegetables
- 1/2–3/4 cup nutritional yeast
- remaining water from the pot
- 1 tbsp. Dijon mustard
- 1 tsp. salt, or to taste
- 1 clove garlic, minced
- 3/4 tsp. turmeric
- pepper, to taste
- optional: a dash of cayenne pepper

Instructions:

1. Boil 2 cups of water.
2. Put in the sweet potato. Leave to boil for 5 minutes.
3. Put in the zucchini, carrots, and onion. Boil for another 5-8 minutes. Remove from heat.
4. Transfer boiled vegetables to a blender.

5. Add the remaining boiled water from the pot.
6. Add in the rest of the ingredients for the cheese sauce and pour over the pasta.
7. Mix until well combined.
8. Serve while warm.

Potato and Egg Salad

Ingredients:

- 800g potato, washed and cut into bite-sized pieces
- 4 large eggs
- 1 red bell pepper, diced
- 160g green beans, cut into small pieces
- 1 small cucumber, cut into sticks
- 3 tbsp. fresh chives, chopped
- 3 tbsp. green tips of scallions or green onions, chopped
- 1 tbsp. lemon juice
- 1 tbsp. wholegrain mustard
- ground black pepper
- 1/3 cup mayonnaise

Instructions:

1. Wash the potatoes over running water and cut them into bite-sized pieces.
2. Fill in a large saucepan with 5 cups of water and add the potatoes.
3. Cook the potatoes over medium-high heat for 15-20 minutes or until soft and tender.
4. Add the green beans and cook for 3-5 minutes. Drain and set aside to cool.
5. Cook the eggs for 10-15 minutes or until hard, then cut into quarters.

6. In a small mixing bowl, mix thoroughly the mayonnaise, lemon juice, wholegrain mustard, and black pepper. This will serve as your salad dressing.
7. Using a large mixing bowl, combine the potatoes, green peas, cucumber, green onions/scallions, red bell peppers, and chives. Add the salad dressing and season with ground black pepper.
8. Mix well and serve.

Avocado Chicken Lemon Salad

Ingredients:

- 2 organic chicken breast, skinless
- curly kale, a bunch, ribs and stems removed
- 1 cup of cooked wheat berries
- 1 ripe avocado, sliced, drizzle it with lemon juice
- 1/2 cup pomegranate arils
- 1/2 cup pine nuts, toasted
- pink peppercorns
- pea shoots

For the rosemary oil marinade:

- 1/2 lemon, zest only
- 1 sprig of rosemary
- 2 tbsp. olive oil
- sea salt
- black pepper

For the lemon vinaigrette:

- 1 tsp. dijon mustard
- 1-2 cloves of garlic, minced
- 2 anchovy fillets, minced
- 1 small lemon, juice only
- 2 tbsp. extra virgin olive oil
- 1/2 tsp. lemon zest
- sea salt

- black pepper

Instructions:

1. Prepare the chicken by washing and draining with a paper towel.
2. Slice through the chicken breasts for the marinade and cook well later.
3. Using a mortar, mix all ingredients for the rosemary oil marinade until you get aromatic oil.
4. Gently rub the chicken with the rosemary oil and marinate for at least 15 minutes at room temperature or up to 8 hours in the refrigerator. Occasionally turn over the bag during the day.
5. Preheat the oven up to 375°F.
6. Heat cast-iron skillet over medium-high heat.
7. Add in chicken breasts. Cook until both sides are brown.
8. Move the skillet to the oven and cook for about 7-10 minutes.
9. Using a whisk, combine all the lemon vinaigrette ingredients in the bowl.
10. Put the kale and lemon vinaigrette in a large mixing bowl. Use your hands to mix for about a minute or two. Adjust seasoning according to your preference.
11. Move kale on a serving plate, topped with avocado slices.

12. Slice the chicken and place it on top of the salad. Top with peppercorns, pomegranate arils, toasted pine nuts, and wheat berries.
13. For garnishing, add pea shoots.
14. Enjoy by serving either warm or chilled, with the grilled lemon on the side.

Guilt-Free Egg Salad

Ingredients:

- 125 ml. mayonnaise, full fat variety
- 6 eggs, hard boiled
- some fresh parsley, chopped
- 1 tsp. curry powder, or to taste

Instructions:

1. Peel the cooked eggs and chop them coarsely. Put the chopped eggs in a large bowl.
2. Add mayonnaise and curry powder into the bowl and blend well.
3. Sprinkle with parsley and serve.

Prosciutto-Roast Beef Tenderloin

Ingredients:

- 4-lb. whole beef tenderloin, tail removed
- 1 tbsp. garlic, finely chopped or crushed
- 1 tbsp. olive oil
- 1/4 tsp. ground black pepper
- 1 tsp. fresh parsley, chopped
- 4 oz. prosciutto, deli-sliced

Instructions:

1. Preheat the oven to 425°F.
2. Place the tenderloin on a chopping board.
3. In a bowl, combine the olive oil, garlic, pepper, and parsley. Rub the garlic mix over the tenderloin.
4. Wrap the tenderloin gently with overlapping prosciutto ribbons until covered. On a roasting pan or cookie sheet, place the tenderloin.
5. Roast until desired doneness is achieved. Roast for 26 to 28 minutes for rare, 30 minutes for medium-rare, and 35 to 40 minutes for well-done.
6. Remove from the oven and allow to rest for 10 minutes before slicing the tenderloin.
7. Serve either cold or warm.

Flavored Italian Meatballs

Ingredients:

- 2/3 lb. lean ground beef
- 1/3 lb. turkey sausage
- 1 shallot, minced
- 2 tbsp. olive oil
- 1 tbsp. garlic clove, minced
- 1/4 cup finely chopped parsley
- 1 tbsp. finely chopped rosemary
- 1 tbsp. thyme, chopped finely
- 1 tbsp. dijon mustard
- 1/4 cup panko bread crumbs
- 2 tbsp. milk
- 1 large egg, beaten

Instructions:

1. Preheat the air-fryer at 400°F.
2. Take a non-stick pan and add oil into it. Heat it over a medium-high flame.
3. Put the shallot in and cook for 2 minutes or until it softens.
4. Add minced garlic and cook for another minute. Remove the pan from the heat.
5. Take a large bowl and add panko crumbs along with milk. Combine and let it stand for 5 minutes.

6. Add the cooked shallot to the panko mixture. Add ground beef, turkey, eggs, thyme, parsley, rosemary, and mustard. Mix them together using a wooden spoon.
7. Take a tablespoon of the mixture and gently shape it into a ball.
8. Keep on making the balls using the mixture.
9. Place them in a single layer over the basket of the air fryer. Cook the meatballs for 10 minutes or until they turn light brown.
10. Serve the meatballs hot.

Chicken Wrap (Cajun Style)

Ingredients:

- keto tortilla
- avocado, half will do, chopped
- cajun chicken
- tomato, chopped
- yogurt, preferably plain or organic, to taste
- lettuce, chopped
- cucumber, chopped
- pepper, to taste
- sea salt, to taste

Instructions:

1. Except for the tortilla, toss all the ingredients for the salad in a bowl.
2. Heat up the tortilla in the microwave for 15 seconds, then plate it nicely.
3. Gently transfer the salad mix to the center of the tortilla. Once done, fold both sides nicely, similar to how a burrito is wrapped.
4. Slice and enjoy eating.

Slow Cooker Dairy-Free Buttered Chicken

Ingredients:

- 2 lbs. boneless and skinless chicken breast, chopped into chunks
- 15 oz. can of full-fat coconut milk
- 15 oz. can of tomato sauce
- 2 tbsp. lemon juice
- 1 cinnamon stick
- 2 tbsp. coconut oil
- 1 tsp. sea salt
- 1 pc. chopped yellow onion
- 5 cloves minced garlic
- 1 tsp chili powder
- 1/2 tsp. cayenne powder
- 1 in. knob ginger, chopped
- 2 tsp. ground turmeric
- 1 tbsp. garam masala
- 1 tbsp. cumin
- 1/2 ground pepper
- 1/2 tsp. ground cinnamon

Instructions:

1. Preheat the skillet and add oil.
2. Sauté onion and garlic for 5 minutes.

3. Add turmeric, garam masala, ginger, salt, pepper, chili powder, cayenne, and cinnamon. Toss to combine all spices. Cook for 1-2 minutes.
4. Transfer the mixture to the slow cooker.
5. Add chicken, coconut milk, lemon juice, tomato sauce, and cinnamon. Cover and cook for 2-3 hours over high heat.
6. Serve hot and garnish with fresh cilantro and some lime juice.

Keto Taco Shells

Ingredients:

- 60 grams of fresh spinach leaves
- 2 eggs
- 1/3 cup almond meal
- 2 tsp psyllium husk
- 1/2 tsp salt
- taco toppings
- smoked chicken
- avocado
- onion
- sour cream
- tomato
- coriander
- chipotle adobo sauce or any low carb sauce

Instruction:

1. Preheat the oven to 160-180°C.
2. Prepare a pan lined with baking paper.
3. Pour the spinach leaves over boiling water and cover for 5 minutes to blanch.
4. Drain and squeeze afterward.
5. Put the spinach into a food processor together with eggs, almond meal, psyllium husk, and salt. Process until fine and smooth.

6. Make 15 cm big circles by placing approximately 1/4 of the mixture onto the pan and spreading it by using a cranked spatula.
7. Afterward, place in the oven and bake for about 9 minutes or until cooked.
8. Set aside to cool and then bake again for another 10 minutes to dry.
9. Once done, fill it with taco toppings and serve.

One-Pot Chicken and Rice

Ingredients:

- 1 lb. boneless skinless chicken thighs, cut into bite-sized chunks
- 2 tbsp. olive oil
- 3 small shallots, diced
- 3 carrots, diced
- 1 cup mushrooms, sliced
- 2 cloves garlic, minced
- 2-1/4 cups chicken broth or stock
- 1-1/2 cups rice, white jasmine rice, rinsed and drained
- 2 tbsp. fresh thyme leaves, chopped
- salt
- pepper

Instructions:

1. Heat olive oil in a Dutch oven over medium heat for a minute.
2. Add chicken and a generous pinch of salt and pepper.
3. Cook for about 7 minutes.
4. Add shallots, mushrooms, and carrots. Cook for another 4 to 5 minutes, stirring frequently.
5. Add garlic, 1 tbsp. thyme, and another pinch of salt and pepper. Cook for another minute.
6. Add chicken stock or broth. Check the taste, and add salt and pepper if preferred.

7. Add rice and bring it to a boil.
8. Reduce heat, stir, cover, and cook for about 20 minutes on low heat.
9. Stir, cover, and remove from heat. Let it sit for about 10 minutes.
10. Fluff rice with a fork and garnish with the remaining fresh thyme.
11. Serve immediately.

Red Velvet Molten Lava Cake

Ingredients:

- 2 tbsp. coconut flour
- 1 tbsp. unsweetened cocoa powder
- 1 tbsp. ground flaxseed meal
- 1/2 tsp. baking powder
- 1/4 tsp. salt
- 1/4 cup 1% milk
- 1/4 tsp. vanilla extract
- 2 eggs
- 1 tsp. chocolate liquid stevia, or 1/2 cup of sugar-free sweetener
- 85% dark chocolate bars, broken into pieces
- 3 drops of red food coloring

Instructions:

1. Mix the coconut flour, cocoa powder, flaxseed, baking powder, and salt.
2. In a separate bowl, whisk the milk, eggs, vanilla extract, stevia, and food coloring together.
3. Pour the dry mixture into the wet mixture. Stir until combined.
4. Adjust food coloring to the redness you desire.
5. Spray oil on a couple of microwave-safe mugs or ramekins.
6. Pour batter into each container.

7. Insert chocolate pieces in the center of each batter.
8. Microwave one cake at a time for about one and a half minutes.
9. Serve and enjoy while warm.

Prevention of Post-Polio Syndrome

PPS cannot be avoided in any known way at this time. Nevertheless, there are measures that you can take to lessen the likelihood that you will develop the condition.

Get vaccinated - Polio is a serious viral infection that can cause paralysis, breathing problems, and even death. Though there is no cure for polio, the disease can be prevented with vaccination. The polio vaccine is safe and effective, and it is the best way to protect yourself from the disease. If you haven't been vaccinated, talk to your doctor about getting the vaccine.

Practice good hygiene - Maintaining a clean and healthy lifestyle is one of the best ways to ward off post-polio syndrome. This necessitates that you wash your hands frequently and abstain from touching any surfaces that could be contaminated. It is critical to protect yourself from potential virus exposure by donning a mask whenever you are in the same room as a sick person.

Don't smoke - Quitting smoking is an essential step in helping to reduce the risk of PPS. Your chances of developing the condition are higher if you are a smoker. If you are a smoker, you should discuss ways to quit with your primary care provider. Taking care of your health, in general, is another important factor in preventing Post-polio Syndrome.

Post-Polio Syndrome and Quality of Life

As a result of post-polio syndrome (PPS), polio survivors frequently suffer from fatigue, muscle weakness, and joint pain. Because of these symptoms, it may be difficult to carry out normal daily activities. On the other hand, there are a number of things that can be done to assist in the management of these symptoms and the improvement of one's quality of life.

First, one must realize the significance of maintaining a healthy diet. Consuming foods that are high in protein but low in fat is one way to help improve muscle strength and decrease feelings of fatigue. In addition to this, it is essential to get the recommended daily allowance of vitamins and minerals and to consume a sufficient amount of water.

Second, regular exercise is necessary for preserving both the function of joints and the strength of muscles. However, it is essential to pay attention to cues from your body and avoid pushing yourself beyond its limits. Exerting yourself beyond your limits can result in fatigue as well as pain.

Last but not least, it is essential to look for support from family, friends, and the resources available in the community. There are a number of organizations that are available to provide assistance and information to people who are coping with PPS. It may be helpful in the management of your symptoms and the improvement of your quality of life to talk to others who are going through the same thing as you are and who understand what you are going through.

PPS can make daily life difficult, but there are a lot of things that can be done to improve the quality of life for people who have the condition. It is possible to manage the symptoms of post-traumatic stress disorder (PPS) and live a full and active life if support is sought out, a healthy diet is adhered to, and regular exercise is performed.

FAQ About Post-Polio Syndrome

What is post-polio syndrome?

Post-polio syndrome (PPS) is a condition that can occur in people who have previously had polio. PPS is characterized by new weakness and muscle pain, as well as fatigue and joint pain. The cause of PPS is unknown, but it is believed to be due to the deterioration of the nerve cells that were damaged by the poliovirus.

How is post-polio syndrome diagnosed?

PPS is typically diagnosed by looking at a person's medical history in conjunction with the symptoms they are experiencing. There is no diagnostic test that is specific to PPS; however, your doctor may order tests to eliminate other potential causes.

What are the symptoms of post-polio syndrome?

The symptoms of PPS can vary from person to person. Common symptoms include new weakness, muscle pain, fatigue, and joint pain. Other symptoms may include difficulty sleeping, trouble swallowing, and depression.

How is post-polio syndrome treated?

There is no cure for PPS, but there are treatments that can help to improve symptoms. Treatment typically focuses on managing pain and fatigue, as well as maintaining muscle strength and joint function.

What is the prognosis for people with post-polio syndrome?

The prognosis for people with PPS is generally good. Most people are able to maintain their quality of life with proper treatment. However, some people may experience a decline in their condition.

Are there any complications of post-polio syndrome?

Complications of PPS can include muscle weakness, joint pain, and fatigue. These symptoms can make it difficult to perform everyday activities. However, there are several things that can be done to help manage these symptoms and improve quality of life.

How can I prevent post-polio syndrome?

There is no known way to prevent PPS. However, early diagnosis and treatment of the condition can help to improve symptoms and quality of life.

What is the long-term outlook for people with post-polio syndrome?

Most people with PPS are able to maintain their quality of life with proper treatment. However, some people may experience a decline in their condition. The long-term outlook for people with PPS is generally good.

Key Takeaways

- Post-polio syndrome (PPS) is a condition that can occur in people who have previously had polio.
- PPS is characterized by new weakness and muscle pain, as well as fatigue and joint pain.
- There is no cure for PPS, but there are treatments that can help to improve symptoms.
- Most people with PPS are able to maintain their quality of life with proper treatment.

References and Helpful Links

Nutrition and post-polio | post polio: Polio place. (n.d.). Retrieved November 12, 2022, from https://www.polioplace.org/living-with-polio/nutrition-and-post-polio#:~:text=I%20now%20eat%20lean%20meat,fortified%20with%20a%20protein%20supplement.

Post-polio syndrome—Diagnosis and treatment—Mayo Clinic. (n.d.). Retrieved November 12, 2022, from https://www.mayoclinic.org/diseases-conditions/post-polio-syndrome/diagnosis-treatment/drc-20355674.

www.ingramcontent.com/pod-product-compliance
Lightning Source LLC
LaVergne TN
LVHW012037060526
838201LV00061B/4656